CW01066968

Keto Vegetarian Cleansing Diet

Lose Weight and Boost Your Energy with Tasty Recipes

Lauren Bellisario

Table of Contents

Zucchini Muffins

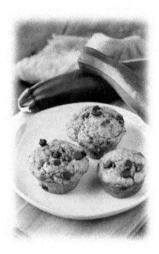

Preparation time: 10 minutes

Cooking time: 35 minutes

Serving: 6

Nutritional Values (Per Serving):

- Calories:137
- Total Fat: 9.5g
- Saturated Fat:4.4 g
- Total Carbs: 3 g
- Dietary Fiber: 0g

- Sugar:1 g
- Protein: 1g
- Sodium: 1001mg

Ingredients:

- ½ cup almond flour
- 1 tsp baking powder
- ½ tsp baking soda
- 1 ½ tsp mustard powder
- Salt and black pepper to taste
- 1/3 cup almond milk
- 1 large egg
- 5 tbsp olive oil
- ½ cup grated cheddar cheese
- 2 zucchinis, grated
- 6 green olives, pitted and sliced
- 1 spring onion, finely chopped
- 1 small red bell pepper, deseeded and chopped
- 1 tbsp freshly chopped thyme

Directions:

1. Preheat the oven to 325 F and grease a pan with cooking spray.

2. In a large bowl, combine the almond flour, baking powder, baking soda, mustard powder, salt, black pepper. In a smaller bowl, whisk the milk, egg, and olive oil. Mix the wet Ingredients into the dry Ingredients and add the cheese, zucchini, olives, spring onion, bell pepper, and thyme. Combine well.

3. Spoon the batter into the muffin holes, ¾-inch full and bake in the oven for 30 to 35 minutes or until golden brown on top and skewer inserted comes out clean.

4. Remove the pan from the oven and allow the muffins to cool in a tin for 10 minutes before removing.

5. Serve immediately for brunch.

Avocado Ricotta Scones

Preparation time: 8 minutes

Cooking time: 25 minutes

Serving: 4

- **Nutritional Values (Per Serving):**
- Calories: 151
- Total Fat: 13.2g
- Saturated Fat:6.8 g
- Total Carbs: 2 g
- Dietary Fiber: 0g
- Sugar: 2g
- Protein:6 g
- Sodium: 126mg

Ingredients:

- 2 cups almond flour 3 tsp baking powder
- ½ cup butter, cold
- 1 cup crumbled ricotta cheese
- 1 ripe avocado, pitted and mashed 1 large egg
- 1/3 cup coconut cream

Directions:

1. Preheat the oven to 350 F and line a baking sheet with parchment paper.
2. In a large bowl, combine the almond flour and baking powder. Add the butter and mix with your hands. Top with the ricotta cheese, avocado, and combine again.
3. Lightly whisk the egg with the coconut cream and slowly stir in the mixture using a fork. Mold 8 to 10 scones out to the batter.
4. Place the scones on the baking sheet and bake in the oven for 20 to 25 minutes or until the scones turn a golden color.
5. Remove; allow cooling for 5 minutes, and serve.

Stewed Tofu with Walnut Cauliflower Grits

Preparation time: 15 minutes

Cooking time: 53 minutes

Serving: 4

Nutritional Values (Per Serving):

- Calories: 651
- Total Fat: 53.9g
- Saturated Fat:23.6 g
- Total Carbs: 19 g
- Dietary Fiber:5 g
- Sugar: 6g
- Protein: 32g
- Sodium:423 mg

Ingredients:

For the stewed tofu:

- 2 tbsp olive oil
- 2 lb tofu, cut into 1-inch cubes
- Salt and black pepper to taste
- 1 large yellow onion, chopped
- 3 garlic cloves, minced
- 2 large tomatoes, diced
- 1 tbsp rosemary
- 1 tbsp smoked paprika
- 2 tsp chili powder
- 2 cups vegetable broth

For the walnut cauliflower grits:

- 2 tbsp butter
- ½ cup walnuts, chopped
- 2 cups cauliflower rice
- ½ cup water
- 1 cup coconut milk
- 1 cup shredded provolone cheese
- Salt to taste

Directions:

For the stewed tofu:

1. Heat the olive oil in a large pot over medium heat, season the tofu with salt and black pepper and cook in the oil until brown, 3 minutes.
2. Stir in the remaining Ingredients and cook over low heat until thickened, 5 to 10 minutes.
3. Adjust the taste with salt and black pepper, and turn the heat off.

For the walnut cauliflower grits:

4. Melt the butter in a medium pot and toast in the walnuts for 5 minutes. Transfer to a cutting board, chop and reserve in a plate.
5. Add the cauliflower rice and water to the pot and cook for 5 minutes or until softened.
6. Stir in the coconut milk, reduce the temperature, and simmer for 3 minutes.
7. Mix in the provolone cheese to melt, fold in the walnuts, and adjust the taste with salt.
8. Spoon the cauliflower grits into serving bowls and top with the stewed tofu.

Tempeh Zucchini Mug Melt

Preparation time: 5 minutes

Cooking time: 2 minutes

Serving: 2

Nutritional Values (Per Serving):

- Calories:136
- Total Fat: 9.6g
- Saturated Fat: 5.2g
- Total Carbs: 5 g
- Dietary Fiber: 2g
- Sugar: 1g
- Protein: 9g
- Sodium: 253mg

Ingredients:

- 4 slices cooked tempeh
- 3 tbsp sour cream

- 1 small zucchini, chopped
- Salt and black pepper to taste
- 2 tbsp chopped green chilies
- 3 oz shredded Monterey Jack cheese

Directions:

1. Divide the tempeh slices in the bottom of two wide mugs and carefully spread with 1 tablespoon of sour cream.
2. Top with the zucchini, season with salt and black pepper, add the green chilies, and top with the remaining sour cream and then the Monterey Jack cheese.
3. Place the mugs in the microwave and cook for 1 to 2 minutes or until the cheese melts.
4. Remove the mugs; allow cooling for 1 minute, and serve.

Vegan Sausage with Vegan Bacon

Preparation time: 5 minutes

Cooking time: 40 minutes

Serving: 4

Nutritional Values (Per Serving):

- Calories:639
- Total Fat: 55.6g
- Saturated Fat:4.6 g
- Total Carbs: 9 g
- Dietary Fiber: 2g
- Sugar: 2g
- Protein:28 g
- Sodium: 999mg

Ingredients:

- 8 large vegan sausages
- ½ cup grated Swiss cheese
- 16 slices vegan bacon
- 1 tsp onion powder
- 1 tsp garlic powder
- Salt and black pepper to taste

Directions:

1. Preheat the oven to 400 F.
2. Cut a slit in the middle of each vegan sausage and stuff evenly with the Swiss cheese. Wrap each vegan sausage with 2 vegan bacon slices each and secure with toothpicks. Season with the onion powder, garlic powder, salt, and black pepper.
3. Place the wrapped vegan sausage on a baking sheet and place in the middle rack of the oven. Cook for 35 to 40 minutes or until the bacon browns and crisps.
4. Remove the food and serve warm with your preferred side dish.

Vegan Sausage Collard Rolls

Preparation time: 10 minutes

Cooking time: 1 hour, 3 minutes, 30 seconds

Servings: 4

Nutritional Values (Per Serving):

- Calories: 356
- Total Fat: 21.2g
- Saturated Fat: 8.8g
- Total Carbs: 10g
- Dietary Fiber: 0g
- Sugar: 3g
- Protein:35 g
- Sodium: 557mg

Ingredients:

- 1 lb crumbled vegan sausages
- 1 tbsp butter

- Salt and black pepper to taste
- 2 tsp coconut aminos
- 1 tsp Dijon mustard
- 1 tsp whole peppercorns
- ¼ tsp cloves
- ¼ tsp allspice
- ½ tsp red pepper flakes
- 1 large bay leaf
- 1 lemon, zested and juiced
- ¼ cup white wine
- ¼ cup freshly brewed coffee
- 2/3 tbsp erythritol
- 8 large Swiss collard leaves
- 1 medium red onion, sliced

Directions:

- In a large pot, add all the Ingredients up to the collard leaves and mix well.
- Close the lid of the pot and cook the Ingredients over low heat for 1 hour or until the vegan sausages cook.
- 10 minutes to the time being up, boil some water in a medium pot over medium heat and add all the collards

with one slice of the onion. Cook for 30 seconds and transfer the leaves immediately to an ice bath to blanch for 5 to 10 minutes.

- Remove the collards, pat dry with a paper towel, and lay flat on a flat surface.
- Divide the vegan sausages mixture onto the collards, top with the onion slices, and roll the leaves over to cover the filling.
- Serve immediately.

Three Cheese Tofu "Meatza"

Preparation time: 10 minutes

Cooking time: 20 minutes

Serving: 4

Nutritional Values (Per Serving):

- Calories:301
- Total Fat: 25.1g
- Saturated Fat: 6.7g
- Total Carbs: 5g
- Dietary Fiber:1 g
- Sugar: 2g
- Protein: 15g
- Sodium: 669mg

Ingredients:

- 1 ½ lb tofu, pressed and crumbled
- Salt and black pepper to taste

- 1 large egg
- 1 tsp thyme
- 3 garlic cloves, minced
- 1 tsp rosemary
- 1 tsp basil
- ½ tbsp oregano
- ¾ cup low-carb tomato sauce
- ¼ cup shredded Pecorino Romano cheese
- 1 cup shredded Monterey Jack cheese
- 1 cup shredded mozzarella cheese

Directions:

1. Preheat the oven to 350 F and lightly grease a medium pizza pan with cooking spray. Set aside.
2. In a large bowl, mix the tofu, salt, black pepper, egg, thyme, garlic, rosemary, basil, and oregano.
3. Transfer the mixture onto the pizza pan and use your hands to flatten the mix onto the pan with 2-inch thickness. Place in the oven and bake for 15 minutes or until the tofu cooks with a light brown crust.
4. Remove the pizza pan and spread the tomato sauce on top.

5. Scatter the three cheeses one after the other on top and bake further in the oven until the cheeses melt, 5 minutes.

6. Remove the "meatza" from the oven, slice, and serve.

Tomatoes and Eggs Plate

Preparation time: 10 minutes

Cooking time: 17 minutes

Serving: 4

Nutritional Values (Per Serving):

- Calories: 501
- Total Fat:43.3 g
- Saturated Fat: 21.5g
- Total Carbs: 17 g
- Dietary Fiber: 5g
- Sugar: 7g
- Protein18: g
- Sodium: 656mg

Ingredients:

- 5 oz vegan bacon, chopped 1 tbsp olive oil
- 8 eggs

- Salt and black pepper to taste
- 1 tbsp butter, room temperature
- ¼ cup red cherry tomatoes
- 2 tbsp chopped fresh oregano

Directions:

1. Cook the vegan bacon in a medium skillet over medium heat until brown and crispy, 5 minutes. Divide onto 4 plates and set aside.
2. Add half of the olive oil into the skillet to heat and crack 4 eggs into the oil. Cook until the egg whites set, but the yolk still runny, 1 minute. Spoon two eggs to the side of the vegan bacon in two plates and fry the remaining eggs using the remaining olive oil. Plate the eggs on two more plates.
3. Melt the butter in the same skillet, cook in the tomatoes until brown around the edges and a bit on the skin, 8 minutes. Add the egg plates.
4. Season the food with salt, black pepper, and garnish with the oregano.
5. Serve warm.

Creamy Cabbage with Tofu and Pine Nuts

Preparation time: 5 minutes

Cooking time: 20 minutes

Serving: 4

Nutritional Values (Per Serving):

- Calories:269
- Total Fat: 21.6g
- Saturated Fat: 7.8g
- Total Carbs: 6g
- Dietary Fiber: 1g
- Sugar: 3g
- Protein: 13g
- Sodium: 298mg

Ingredients:

For the fried tofu:

- 2 tbsp butter
- 25 oz tofu, cut into 6 slabs

For the creamy cabbage:

- 2 oz butter
- 25 oz green canon cabbage, shredded
- 1 ¼ cups heavy cream
- ½ cup chopped fresh marjoram
- Salt and black pepper to taste
- ½ lemon, zested
- 2 tbsp toasted pine nuts

Directions:

For the fried tofu:

1. Melt the butter in a medium skillet over medium heat and fry the tofu on both sides until lightly brown on the outside, 10 minutes. Transfer to a plate and keep warm until ready to serve.

For the creamy cabbage:

1. Melt the butter in the skillet and sauté the cabbage while occasionally stirring until the cabbage turns golden brown, 4 minutes.
2. Mix in the heavy cream, allow bubbling, and season with the marjoram, salt, black pepper, and lemon zest.
3. Divide the tofu onto four plates, spoon the cabbage to the side of the tofu, and sprinkle the pine nuts on the cabbage.
4. Serve warm.

Tempeh Mushroom Omelet

Preparation time: 10 minutes

Cooking time: 20 minutes

Serving: 2

Nutritional Values (Per Serving):

- Calories:355
- Total Fat:29.9 g
- Saturated Fat:12.5 g
- Total Carbs: 4 g
- Dietary Fiber: 0 g
- Sugar: g
- Protein: 18g
- Sodium: 324mg

Ingredients:

- 2 tbsp olive oil
- 2 oz tempeh, crumbled

- Salt and black pepper to taste
- 1 small white onion, chopped
- ¼ cup sliced cremini mushrooms
- 2 tbsp butter
- 6 eggs
- 2 oz shredded cheddar cheese

Directions:

1. Heat half of the olive oil in a medium frying pan, add the tempeh, season with salt and black pepper, and fry until brown, 10 minutes. Transfer to a plate and set aside.
2. Heat the remaining olive oil in the pan and sauté the onion and mushrooms until softened, 8 minutes. Spoon to the side of the tempeh and set aside.
3. Melt the butter in the pan over low heat.
4. Beat the eggs with some salt, black pepper, and pour into the pan. Swirl to spread the egg around the pan and once the omelet begins to firm, top with the tempeh, mushroom-onion mixture, and cheddar cheese.
5. Use a spatula to carefully release the egg from around the edges of the pan and flip the egg over the stuffing.
6. Once beneath the eggs start to golden brown, 2 minutes, slide the eggs onto a serving plate.
7. Using a knife, divide into half and serve warm.

Mushrooms and Radishes Mix

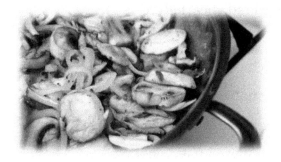

Preparation time: 10 minutes

Cooking time: 25 minutes

Servings: 4

Nutritional Values (Per Serving):

- Calories 182
- Fat 4
- Fiber 2
- Carbs 6
- Protein 8

Ingredients:

- 1 pound white mushrooms, halved
- ½ pound radishes, halved
- 4 scallions, chopped
- 4 garlic cloves, minced
- 2 tablespoons olive oil
- ½ cup veggie stock
- 2 tablespoons parsley, chopped
- 1 teaspoon coriander, ground
- 1 teaspoon rosemary, dried
- A pinch of salt and black pepper

Directions:

1. Heat up a pan with the oil over medium heat, add the scallions, garlic, coriander and rosemary, stir and cook for 5 minutes.
2. Add the mushrooms, radishes and the other ingredients, toss, cook over medium heat for 20 minutes, divide between plates and serve as a side dish.

Sesame and Chives Rice

Preparation time: 10 minutes

Cooking time: 25 minutes

Servings: 4

Nutritional Values (Per Serving):

- Calories 261
- Fat 6
- Fiber 8
- Carbs 10
- Protein 6

Ingredients:

- 2 tablespoons olive oil
- 1 cup cauliflower rice
- 1 cup veggie stock
- 2 tablespoon shallots, chopped
- 2 tablespoons chives, chopped

- 1 teaspoon sesame seeds, toasted
- A pinch of salt and black pepper

Directions:

1. Heat up a pan with the oil over medium heat, add the shallots and chives and sauté for 5 minutes.
2. Add the cauliflower rice and the other ingredients, toss, cook over medium heat for 20 minutes more, divide between plates and serve.

Mashed Broccoli

Preparation time: 10 minutes

Cooking time: 25 minutes

Servings: 4

Nutritional Values (Per Serving):

- Calories 200
- Fat 4
- Fiber 4
- Carbs 7
- Protein 10

Ingredients:

- 1 and ½ cups water
- 1 pound broccoli florets
- 2 teaspoons olive oil
- A pinch of salt and black pepper
- ½ teaspoon turmeric powder

- ½ teaspoon cumin, ground
- 1 tablespoon chives, chopped

Directions:

1. Put the water in a pot, add the broccoli, salt and pepper, bring to a boil and cook over medium heat for 25 minutes.
2. Drain the broccoli, transfer to a bowl, and mash using a potato masher.
3. Add the rest of the ingredients, mash everything again, stir as well, divide between plates and serve as a side dish.

Balsamic Hot Radishes

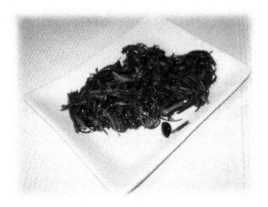

Preparation time: 10 minutes

Cooking time: 20 minutes

Servings: 4

Nutritional Values (Per Serving):

- Calories 182
- Fat 5
- Fiber 5
- Carbs 9
- Protein 9

Ingredients:

- 2 tablespoons avocado oil
- 1 pound radishes, halved
- 1 tablespoon balsamic vinegar
- A pinch of salt and black pepper
- A pinch of chili powder

Directions:

1. Heat up a pan with the oil over medium heat, add the radishes, vinegar and the other ingredients, toss, cook for 20 minutes, divide between plates and serve as a side dish.

Turmeric Coconut Rice Mix

Preparation time: 10 minutes

Cooking time: 20 minutes

Servings: 4

Nutritional Values (Per Serving):

- Calories 211
- Fat 5
- Fiber 4
- Carbs 6
- Protein 12

Ingredients:

- 1 cup cauliflower rice
- 1 tablespoon coconut cream
- 1 cup coconut milk
- A pinch of salt and black pepper
- 1 teaspoon turmeric powder

- ½ teaspoon garam masala
- 1 tablespoon cilantro, chopped

Directions:

1. Put the coconut milk in a pan, heat up over medium heat, add the rice, cream and the other ingredients, toss, cook for 20 minutes, divide between plates and serve.

Wild Mushrooms and Radish Rice

Preparation time: 10 minutes

Cooking time: 25 minutes

Servings: 4

Nutritional Values (Per Serving):

- Calories 189
- Fat 3
- Fiber 4
- Carbs 9
- Protein 8

Ingredients:

- 2 cups cauliflower rice
- 2 tablespoons avocado oil
- ½ cup wild mushrooms, sliced

- ½ cup radishes, halved
- 3 shallots, chopped
- 1 cup veggie stock
- 1 teaspoon fennel seeds
- 1 teaspoon coriander, ground
- A pinch of salt and black pepper
- 2 tablespoons chives, chopped

Directions:

2. Heat up a pan with the oil over medium heat, add the shallots and the mushrooms and sauté for 5 minutes.
3. Add the cauliflower rice, the radishes and the other ingredients, toss, cook over medium heat for 20 minutes, divide between plates and serve as a side dish.

Roasted Radishes

Preparation time: 10 minutes

Cooking time: 35 minutes

Servings: 2

Nutritional Values (Per Serving):

- Calories – 122
- Fat – 12
- Fiber – 1
- Carbs – 3
- Protein - 14

Ingredients:

- 2 cups radishes, cut in quarters
- Salt and ground black pepper, to taste
- 2 tablespoons butter, melted

- 1 tablespoon fresh chives, chopped
- 1 tablespoon lemon zest

Directions:

1. Spread the radishes on a lined baking sheet.
2. Add the salt, pepper, chives, lemon zest, and butter, toss to coat, and bake in the oven at 375°F for 35 minutes.
3. Divide on plates and serve.

Crispy Radishes

Preparation time: 10 minutes

Cooking time: 20 minutes

Servings: 4

Nutritional Values (Per Serving):

- Calories – 30
- Fat – 1
- Fiber - 0. 4
- Carbs – 1
- Protein - 0. 1

Ingredients:

- Vegetable oil cooking spray
- 15 radishes, sliced
- Salt and ground black pepper, to taste
- 1 tablespoon fresh chives, chopped

Directions:

1. Arrange the radish slices on a lined baking sheet and spray them with cooking oil.
2. Season with salt and pepper, sprinkle with the chives, place in an oven at 375°F, and bake for 10 minutes.
3. Flip them and bake for 10 minutes.
4. Serve cold.

Creamy Radishes

Preparation time: 10 minutes

Cooking time: 25 minutes

Servings: 1

Nutritional Values (Per Serving):

- Calories – 340
- Fat – 23
- Fiber – 3
- Carbs – 6
- Protein - 15

Ingredients:

- 7 ounces radishes, cut in half
- 2 tablespoons sour cream
- 2 bacon slices
- 1 tablespoon green onion, peeled and chopped
- 1 tablespoon cheddar cheese, grated

- Hot sauce, to taste
- Salt and ground black pepper, to taste

Directions:

1. Put the radishes into a pot, add the water to cover, bring to a boil over medium heat, cook them for 10 minutes, and drain.
2. Heat up a pan over medium-high heat, add the bacon, cook until crispy, transfer to paper towels, drain the grease, crumble, and leave aside.
3. Return the pan to medium heat, add the radishes, stir, and sauté them for 7 minutes.
4. Add the onion, salt, pepper, hot sauce, and sour cream, stir, and cook for 7 minutes.
5. Transfer to a plate, top with crumbled bacon and cheddar cheese, and serve.

Radish Soup

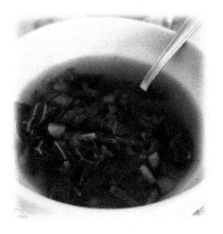

Preparation time: 10 minutes

Cooking time: 20 minutes

Servings: 4

Nutritional Values (Per Serving):

- Calories – 120
- Fat – 2
- Fiber – 1
- Carbs – 3
- Protein - 10

Ingredients:

- 2 bunches radishes, cut in quarters
- Salt and ground black pepper, to taste
- 6 cups chicken stock
- 2 stalks celery, chopped
- 3 tablespoons coconut oil
- 6 garlic cloves, peeled and minced
- 1 onion, peeled and chopped

Directions:

1. Heat up a pot with the oil over medium heat, add the onion, celery, and garlic, stir, and cook for 5 minutes.
2. Add the radishes, stock, salt, and pepper, stir, bring to a boil, cover, and simmer for 15 minutes.
3. Divide into soup bowls and serve.

Avocado Salad

Preparation time: 10 minutes

Cooking time: 0 minutes

Servings: 4

Nutritional Values (Per Serving):

- Calories – 100
- Fat – 10
- Fiber – 2
- Carbs – 5
- Protein - 8

Ingredients:

- 2 avocados, pitted, and mashed
- Salt and ground black pepper, to taste
- ¼ teaspoon lemon stevia
- 1 tablespoon white vinegar
- 14 ounces coleslaw mix

- Juice from 2 limes
- ¼ cup onion, chopped
- ¼ cup fresh cilantro, chopped
- 2 tablespoons olive oil

Directions:

1. Put the coleslaw mixture in a salad bowl.
2. Add the avocado mash and onions, and toss to coat.
3. In a bowl, mix the lime juice with salt, pepper, oil, vinegar, and stevia, and stir well.
4. Add this to salad, toss to coat, sprinkle cilantro, and serve.

Avocado and Egg Salad

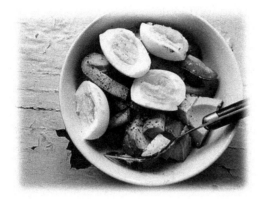

Preparation time: 10 minutes

Cooking time: 7 minutes

Servings: 4

Nutritional Values (Per Serving):

- Calories – 234
- Fat – 12
- Fiber – 4
- Carbs – 7
- Protein - 12

Ingredients:

- 4 cups mixed lettuce leaves, torn
- 4 eggs
- 1 avocado, pitted, and sliced
- ¼ cup mayonnaise
- 2 teaspoons mustard
- 2 garlic cloves, peeled and minced
- 1 tablespoon fresh chives, chopped
- Salt and ground black pepper, to taste

Directions:

1. Put water in a pot, add some salt, add the eggs, bring to a boil over medium-high heat, boil for 7 minutes, drain, cool, peel, and chop them. In a salad bowl, mix the lettuce with eggs, and avocado.
2. Add the chives and garlic, some salt, and pepper, and toss to coat.
3. In a bowl, mix the mustard with mayonnaise, salt, and pepper, and stir well.
4. Add this to the salad, toss well, and serve.

Chickpea, Tomato, And Eggplant Stew

Preparation time: 5 Minutes

Cooking time: 55 Minutes

Servings: 4

Ingredients:

- 1 tablespoon olive oil
- 1 large onion, chopped
- 1 medium eggplant, peeled and cut into ½-inch dice
- 2 medium carrots, cut into ¼-inch slices
- 1 large Yukon Gold potato, peeled and cut into ½-inch dice
- 1 medium red bell pepper, cut into 1-inch dice
- 3 garlic cloves, minced
- 2 cups cooked or 1 (15.5-ounce) cans chickpeas, drained and rinsed if canned

- 1 (28-ounce) can diced tomatoes, undrained
- 1 tablespoon minced fresh parsley
- 1/2 teaspoon dried oregano
- 1/2 teaspoon dried basil
- 1 tablespoon soy sauce
- 1/2 cup vegetable broth, or water
- Salt and freshly ground black pepper

Directions:

1. In a large saucepan, heat the oil over medium heat. Add the onion, eggplant, and carrots, cover, and cook until vegetables begin to soften, about 5 minutes.
2. Reduce heat to low. Add the potato, bell pepper, and garlic and cook, stirring, uncovered, for 5 minutes. Stir in the chickpeas, tomatoes, parsley, oregano, basil, soy sauce, and broth. Season with salt and black pepper to taste. Cover and cook until vegetables are tender, about 45 minutes. Serve immediately.

Tomato Cream Pasta (Pressure Cooker)

Nutrition per Serving

- Calories: 321
- Protein: 14g
- Total fat: 3g
- Saturated fat: 0g
- Carbohydrates: 16g
- Fiber: 9g

Ingredients:

- 1 (28-ounce) can crushed tomatoes
- 1 tablespoon dried basil
- ½ teaspoon garlic powder
- 10 ounces whole-grain pasta
- ½ teaspoon salt, plus more as needed
- 1½ cups water or unsalted vegetable broth
- 1 cup unsweetened nondairy milk or creamer

- 2 cups chopped fresh spinach (optional)
- Freshly ground black pepper

Directions:

1. Preparing the ingredients. In your electric pressure cooker's cooking pot, combine the tomatoes, basil, garlic powder, pasta, salt, and water.

2. High pressure for 4 minutes. Close and lock the lid and ensure the pressure valve is sealed, then select High Pressure and set the time for 4 minutes.

3. Pressure Release. Once the cook time is complete, let the pressure release naturally for 5 minutes, then quick release any remaining pressure, being careful not to get your fingers or face near the steam release. Once all the pressure has released, carefully unlock and remove the lid.

4. Stir in the milk and spinach (if using). Taste and season with more salt, if needed, and pepper. On your pressure cooker, select Sauté or Simmer. Let cook for 4 to 5 minutes, until the sauce thickens and the greens wilt.

Senegalese Soup

Preparation time: 5 Minutes

Cooking time: 40 Minutes

Servings: 4

Ingredients:

- 1 tablespoon canola or grapeseed oil
- 1 medium onion, chopped
- 1 medium carrot, chopped
- 1 garlic clove, minced
- 3 Granny Smith apples, peeled, cored, and chopped
- 2 tablespoons hot or mild curry powder
- 2 teaspoons tomato paste
- 3 cups light vegetable broth (homemade, store-bought or water)
- Salt
- 1 cup plain unsweetened soy milk
- 4 teaspoons mango chutney, homemade or store-bought, for garnish

Directions:

1. In a large soup pot, heat the oil over medium heat. Add the onion, carrot, and garlic. Cover and cook until softened, about 10 minutes. Add the apples and continue to cook, uncovered, stirring occasionally, until the apples begin to soften, about 5 minutes. Add the curry powder and cook, stirring, 1 minute. Stir in the tomato paste, broth, and salt to taste. Simmer, uncovered, for 30 minutes.

2. Puree the soup in the pot with an immersion blender or in a blender or food processor, in batches if necessary. Pour the soup into a large container, stir in the soy milk, cover, and refrigerate until chilled, about 3 hours.

3. Ladle the soup into bowls, garnish each with a teaspoonful of chutney, and serve.

Delicious Sambal Seitan Noodles

Preparation time: 60 minutes

Serving: 4

Nutritional Values (Per Serving):

- Calories:538
- Total Fat:41.1g
- Saturated Fat:16.2g
- Total Carbs:20g
- Dietary Fiber:14g
- Sugar:5g
- Protein:29g
- Sodium:640mg

Ingredients:

For the shirataki noodles:

- 2 (8 oz) packs Miracle noodles, garlic and herb
- Salt to season

For the sambal seitan:

- 1 tbsp olive oil
- 1 lb seitan
- 4 garlic cloves, minced
- 1-inch ginger, peeled and grated
- 1 tsp liquid erythritol
- 1 tbsp sugar-free tomato paste
- 2 fresh basil leaves + extra for garnishing
- 2 tbsp sambal oelek
- 2 tbsp plain vinegar
- 1 cup water
- 2 tbsp coconut aminos
- Salt to taste
- 1 tbsp unsalted butter

Directions:

For the shirataki noodles:

1. Bring 2 cups of water to a boil in a medium pot over medium heat.
2. Strain the Miracle noodles through a colander and rinse very well under hot running water.
3. Allow proper draining and pour the noodles into the boiling water. Cook for 3 minutes and strain again.
4. Place a dry skillet over medium heat and stir-fry the shirataki noodles until visibly dry, 1 to 2 minutes. Season with salt, plate and set aside.

For the seitan sambal:

5. Heat the olive oil in a large pot and cook in the seitan until brown, 5 minutes.
6. Stir in the garlic, ginger, liquid erythritol and cook for 1 minute.
7. Add the tomato paste, cook for 2 minutes and mix in the basil, sambal oelek, vinegar, water, coconut aminos, and salt. Cover the pot and continue cooking over low heat for 30 minutes.
8. Uncover, add the shirataki noodles, butter and mix well into the sauce.

Spinach and Pomegranate Salad

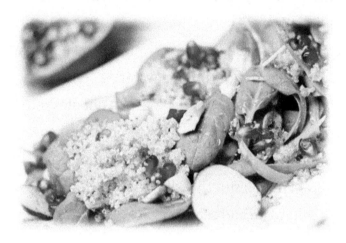

Preparation time: 10 Minutes

Cooking time: 0 Minutes

Servings: 4

Ingredients:

- 10 ounces baby spinach
- seeds from 1 pomegranate
- 1 cup fresh blackberries

- ¼ red onion, thinly sliced
- ½ cup chopped pecans
- ¼ cup balsamic vinegar
- ¾ cup olive oil
- ½ teaspoon sea salt
- ½ teaspoon freshly ground black pepper

Directions:

1. In a large bowl, combine the spinach, pomegranate seeds, blackberries, red onion, and pecans.
2. In a small bowl, whisk together the vinegar, olive oil, salt, and pepper. Toss with the salad and serve immediately.

Cobb Salad with Portobello Bacon

Preparation time: 15 Minutes

Cooking time: 0 Minutes

Servings: 4

Ingredients:

- 2 heads romaine lettuce, finely chopped
- 1 pint cherry tomatoes, halved
- 1 avocado, peeled, pitted, and diced
- 1 cup frozen (and thawed) or fresh corn kernels
- 1 large cucumber, peeled and diced
- Portobello Bacon or store-bought vegan bacon
- 4 scallions, thinly sliced
- Unhidden Valley Ranch Dressing or store-bought vegan ranch dressing

Directions:

1. Scatter a layer of romaine in the bottom of each of 4 salad bowls. With the following ingredients, create lines that cross the top of the romaine, in this order: tomatoes, avocado, corn, cucumber, and portobello bacon.
2. Sprinkle with the scallions and drizzle with ranch dressing.

German-Style Potato Salad

Preparation time: 15 Minutes

Cooking time: 0 Minutes

Servings: 4 To 6

Ingredients:

- 1½ pounds white potatoes, unpeeled
- ½ cup olive oil
- 4 slices tempeh bacon, homemade or store-bought
- 1 medium bunch green onions, chopped
- 1 tablespoon whole-wheat flour
- 2 tablespoons sugar
- ⅓ cup white wine vinegar
- ¼ cup water
- ½ teaspoon salt
- ⅛ teaspoon freshly ground black pepper

Directions:

1. In a large pot of boiling salted water, cook the potatoes until just tender, about 30 minutes. Drain well and set aside to cool.

2. In a large skillet, heat the oil over medium heat. Add the tempeh bacon and cook until browned on both sides, about 5 minutes total. Remove from skillet, and set aside to cool.

3. Cut the cooled potatoes into 1-inch chunks and place in a large bowl. Crumble or chop the cooked tempeh bacon and add to the potatoes.

4. Reheat the skillet over medium heat. Add the green onions and cook for 1 minute to soften. Stir in the flour, sugar, vinegar, water, salt, and pepper, and bring to a boil, stirring until smooth. Pour the hot dressing onto the potatoes. Stir gently to combine and serve.

Sweet Pearl Couscous Salad with Pear & Cranberries

Preparation time: 5 Minutes

Cooking time: 10 Minutes

Servings: 4

Nutrition per Serving:

- Calories: 365
- Protein: 6g
- Total fat: 14g
- Saturated fat: 2g
- Carbohydrates: 55g
- Fiber: 4g

Ingredients:

- 1 cup pearl couscous
- 1½ cups water

- Salt
- ¼ cup olive oil
- ¼ cup freshly squeezed orange juice
- 1 tablespoon sugar, maple syrup, or Simple Syrup
- 1 pear, cored and diced
- ½ cucumber, diced
- ¼ cup dried cranberries or raisins

Directions:

1. In a small pot, combine the couscous, water, and a pinch of salt. Bring to a boil over high heat, turn the heat to low, and cover the pot. Simmer for about 10 minutes, until the couscous is al dente.
2. Meanwhile, in a large bowl, whisk together the olive oil, orange juice, and sugar. Season to taste with salt and whisk again to combine.
3. Add the pear, cucumber, cranberries, and cooked couscous. Toss to combine. Store leftovers in an airtight container in the refrigerator for up to 1 week.

Strawberry Shortcake Chaffle Bowls

Preparation time: 10 minutes

Cooking time: 28 minutes

Servings: 4

Nutritional Values (Per Serving):

- Calories 235
- Fats 20.62g
- Carbs 5.9g
- Net Carbs 5g
- Protein 7.51g

Ingredients:

- 1 egg, beaten

- ½ cup finely grated mozzarella cheese
- 1 tbsp almond flour
- ¼ tsp baking powder
- 2 drops cake batter extract
- 1 cup cream cheese, softened
- 1 cup fresh strawberries, sliced
- 1 tbsp sugar-free maple syrup

Directions:

1. Preheat the cast iron pan.
2. Meanwhile, in a medium bowl, whisk all the ingredients except the cream cheese and strawberries.
3. Open the iron, pour in half of the mixture, cover, and cook until crispy, 6 to 7 minutes.
4. Remove the chaffle bowl onto a plate and set aside.
5. Make a second chaffle bowl with the remaining batter.
6. To serve, divide the cream cheese into the chaffle bowls and top with the strawberries.
7. Drizzle the filling with the maple syrup and serve.

Chaffles with Raspberry Syrup

Preparation time: 10 minutes

Cooking time: 38 minutes

Servings: 4

Nutritional Values (Per Serving):

- Calories 105
- Fats 7.11g
- Carbs 4.31g
- Net Carbs 2.21g
- Protein 5.83g

Ingredients:

For the chaffles:

- 1 egg, beaten
- ½ cup finely shredded cheddar cheese
- 1 tsp almond flour
- 1 tsp sour cream

For the raspberry syrup:

- 1 cup fresh raspberries
- ¼ cup swerve sugar
- ¼ cup water
- 1 tsp vanilla extract

Directions:

For the chaffles:

1. Preheat the cast iron pan.
2. Meanwhile, in a medium bowl, mix the egg, cheddar cheese, almond flour, and sour cream.
3. Open the iron, pour in half of the mixture, cover, and cook until crispy, 7 minutes.
4. Remove the chaffle onto a plate and make another with the remaining batter. For the raspberry syrup:
5. Meanwhile, add the raspberries, swerve sugar, water, and vanilla extract to a medium pot. Set over low heat and cook until the raspberries soften and sugar becomes syrupy. Occasionally stir while mashing the raspberries as you go. Turn the heat off when your desired consistency is achieved and set aside to cool.
6. Drizzle some syrup on the chaffles and enjoy when ready.

Chaffle Cannoli

Preparation time: 15 minutes

Cooking time: 28 minutes

Servings: 4

Nutritional Values (Per Serving):

- Calories 308
- Fats 25.05g
- Carbs 5.17g
- Net Carbs 5.17g
- Protein 15.18g

Ingredients:

For the chaffles:

- 1 large egg
- 1 egg yolk
- 3 tbsp butter, melted
- 1 tbso swerve confectioner's
- 1 cup finely grated Parmesan cheese

- 2 tbsp finely grated mozzarella cheese

For the cannoli filling:

- ½ cup ricotta cheese
- 2 tbsp swerve confectioner's sugar
- 1 tsp vanilla extract
- 2 tbsp unsweetened chocolate chips for garnishing

Directions:

1. Preheat the cast iron pan.
2. Meanwhile, in a medium bowl, mix all the ingredients for the chaffles.
3. Open the iron, pour in a quarter of the mixture, cover, and cook until crispy, 7 minutes.
4. Remove the chaffle onto a plate and make 3 more with the remaining batter.
5. Meanwhile, for the cannoli filling:
6. Beat the ricotta cheese and swerve confectioner's sugar until smooth. Mix in the vanilla.
7. On each chaffle, spread some of the filling and wrap over.
8. Garnish the creamy ends with some chocolate chips.
9. Serve immediately.

Roasted Almonds

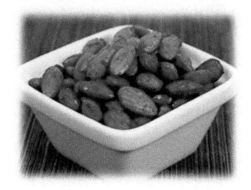

Preparation time: 10 minutes

Cooking time: 10 minutes

Servings: 8

Nutritional Values (per Serving):

- Calories 150
- Fat 13.3 g
- Carbohydrates 5.1 g
- Sugar 1 g
- Protein 5 g
- Cholesterol 4 mg

Ingredients:

- 2 cups almonds
- ¼ tsp chili powder
- 1 tbsp butter, melted
- Salt

Directions:

1. Preheat the air fryer to 330 F.
2. Add almonds, chili powder, butter, and salt into the bowl and toss well.
3. Add almonds into the air fryer basket and cook for 10 minutes. Toss after every 3 minutes.
4. Serve and enjoy.

Crispy Onion Fritters

Preparation time: 10 minutes

Cooking time: 12 minutes

Servings: 4

Nutritional Values (per Serving):

- Calories 333
- Fat 10.5 g
- Carbohydrates 49.7 g
- Sugar 7.1 g
- Protein 11.3 g
- Cholesterol 1 mg

Ingredients:

- 1 onion, sliced
- 2 tbsp olive oil
- ½ tbsp green chili paste
- ½ cup rice flour

- 1 cup chickpea flour
- ¼ tsp turmeric
- Pinch of baking soda
- Salt
- Water

Directions:

1. Add all ingredients except water into the bowl and mix until well combined. Slowly add water and mix until crumbly batter is formed.
2. Preheat the air fryer to 350 F.
3. Spray air fryer basket with cooking spray.
4. Make the medium size of fritters from the mixture and place into the air fryer basket and cook for 12 minutes. Flip fritters halfway through.
5. Serve and enjoy.

Spicy Chickpeas

Preparation time: 10 minutes

Cooking time: 30 minutes

Servings: 6

Nutritional Values (per Serving):

- Calories 235
- Fat 3.8 g
- Carbohydrates 40 g
- Sugar 6.2 g
- Protein 11.2 g
- Cholesterol 0 mg

Ingredients:

- 30 oz can chickpeas, drained
- ½ tsp chili powder
- ¼ tsp cayenne

- 2 tbsp olive oil
- Salt

Directions:

1. Preheat the air fryer to 350 F.
2. In a bowl, toss chickpeas with oil and salt.
3. Add chickpeas into the air fryer basket and cook for 30 minutes. Shake basket halfway through.
4. Transfer chickpeas into the bowl. Add chili powder and cayenne and toss well.
5. Serve and enjoy.

Green Tea Coconut Cake

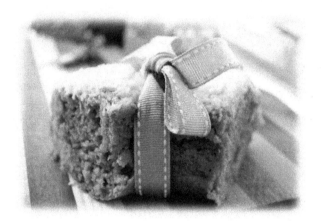

Preparation time: 10 minutes

Cooking time: 35 minutes

Servings: 6

Nutritional Values (Per Serving):

- Calories 484
- Fat 30.7
- Fiber 26.5

- Carbs 46.5
- Protein 10.4

Ingredients:

- 2 tablespoons green tea powder
- 2 cups warm coconut milk
- ½ cup coconut cream
- 3 tablespoons avocado oil
- 1 cup stevia
- 3 tablespoons flaxseed mixed with 4 tablespoons water
- 2 teaspoons vanilla extract
- 3 cups coconut flour
- 1 teaspoon baking soda
- teaspoon baking powder

Directions:

1. In a bowl, combine the green tea powder with the coconut milk, the cream and the other ingredients and whisk well.

2. Pour this into a cake pan lined with parchment paper, introduce in the oven at 370 degrees F and bake for 35 minutes.

3. Leave the cake to cool down, slice and serve.

Grapes Vanilla Cream

Preparation time: 1 hour

Cooking time: 0 minutes

Servings: 4

Nutritional Values (Per Serving):

- Calories 432
- Fat 43
- Fiber 4.2
- Carbs 14
- Protein 4.3

Ingredients:

- 2 cups almond milk
- 1 cup grapes, halved
- 1 cup coconut cream
- 3 tablespoons stevia

- 1 teaspoon vanilla extract
- 1 teaspoon gelatin powder

Directions:

In a bowl, combine the grapes with the coconut cream, the almond milk and the other ingredients, whisk well, divide into cups and keep in the fridge for 1 hour before serving.

Grapes Pie

Preparation time: 10 minutes

Cooking time: 40 minutes

Servings: 6

Nutritional Values (Per Serving):

- Calories 200
- Fat 4.4
- Fiber 3
- Carbs 7.6
- Protein 8

Ingredients:

- ½ cup stevia
- 2 cups grapes, halved
- ½ teaspoon vanilla extract
- 1 cup coconut flour
- 1 teaspoon baking powder

- ½ cup coconut cream
- 3 tablespoons flaxseed mixed with 4 tablespoons water

Directions:

1. In a bowl, combine the grapes with the stevia, vanilla and the other ingredients, whisk well and pour into a pie pan.
2. Bake at 375 digress F for 40 minutes, cool down, slice and serve.

Berry Cream

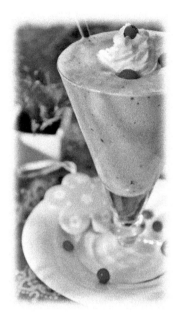

Preparation time: 2 hours

Cooking time: 0 minutes

Servings: 4

Nutritional Values (Per Serving):

- Calories 200
- Fat 4.5

- Fiber 3.3
- Carbs 5.6
- Protein 3.4

Ingredients:

- 1 cup strawberries, chopped
- 1 cup blueberries
- 1 cup coconut cream
- 1/3 cup stevia
- 1 teaspoon lime juice
- ¼ teaspoon nutmeg, ground
- ½ teaspoon vanilla extract

Directions:

1. In a blender, combine the strawberries with the blueberries and the other ingredients, pulse well, divide into cups and keep in the fridge for 2 hours before serving.

Cold Grapes and Avocado Cream

Preparation time: 1 hour

Cooking time: 0 minutes

Servings: 4

Nutritional Values (Per Serving):

- Calories 152
- Fat 4.4
- Fiber 5.5
- Carbs 5.1
- Protein 0.8

Ingredients:

- ½ cup stevia
- 2 cups grapes, halved
- 1 avocado, peeled, pitted and chopped
- 1 cup almond milk
- Zest of 1 lime, grated

- ½ cup coconut cream

Directions:

1. In a blender, combine the grapes with the avocado and the other ingredients, pulse well, divide into bowls and keep in the fridge for 1 hour before serving.

Lime Plum Cake

Preparation time: 10 minutes

Cooking time: 40 minutes

Servings: 4

Nutritional Values (Per Serving):

- Calories 209
- Fat 6.4
- Fiber 6
- Carbs 8
- Protein 6.6

Ingredients:

- 2 cups coconut flour
- 1 tablespoon flaxseed mixed with 2 tablespoons water
- 5 tablespoons stevia
- 1 and ½ cups almond milk
- 2 pounds plums, pitted and chopped

- Juice of ½ lime
- Zest of 1 lime, grated
- 1 teaspoon baking powder

Directions:

1. In a bowl, combine the coconut flour with the flaxseed mix, the plums and the other ingredients and whisk well.
2. Pour the cake mix into a cake pan lined with parchment paper, spread, introduce in the oven and bake at 350 degrees F for 40 minutes.
3. Cool down, slice and serve.

Avocado Cookies

Preparation time: 10 minutes

Cooking time: 20 minutes

Servings: 10

Nutritional Values (Per Serving):

- Calories 200
- Fat 4.5
- Fiber 3.4
- Carbs 9.5
- Protein 2.4

Ingredients:

- 1 cup avocado, peeled, pitted and mashed
- 2 cups coconut flour
- 2 tablespoons flaxseed mixed with 3 tablespoons water
- 1 teaspoon vanilla extract
- 1 teaspoon baking powder

- 1 cup avocado oil
- ½ cup stevia
- 1 cup coconut, unsweetened and shredded

Directions:

1. In a bowl, combine the flour with the avocado, the flaxseed and the other ingredients, and whisk really well.
2. Scoop tablespoons of dough on a baking sheet lined with parchment paper, flatten them, introduce them in the oven at 350 degrees F and bake for 20 minutes.
3. Leave the cookies to cool down and serve.

Blackberries Brownies

Preparation time: 10 minutes

Cooking time: 20 minutes

Servings: 8

Nutritional Values (Per Serving):

- Calories 200
- Fat 4.5
- Fiber 2.
- Carbs 8.7
- Protein 4.3

Ingredients:

- 1 cup almond flour
- 1 cup blackberries
- 1 tablespoon stevia
- 1 avocado, peeled, pitted and chopped
- ½ teaspoon baking soda

- 4 tablespoons coconut oil, melted
- 2 tablespoons lime zest, grated
- Cooking spray

Directions:

1. In a food processor, combine the flour with the blackberries and the other ingredients except the cooking spray and pulse well.
2. Pour this into a pan greased with cooking spray, spread evenly, introduce in the oven at 380 degrees F and bake for 20 minutes.
3. Cut the brownies and serve cold.

Raspberry Protein Shake (vegan)

Preparation time: 5 minutes

Cooking time: 0 minute

Servings: 2

Nutritions:

- Calories: 311kcal
- Net carbs: 4.6g
- Fat: 25.7g
- Protein: 14.65g
- Fiber: 3.5g
- Sugar: 3.35g

Ingredients:

- 1 cup full-fat coconut milk (or alternatively, use almond milk)
- Optional: ¼ cup coconut cream
- 1 scoop organic soy protein (chocolate or vanilla flavor)
- ½ cup raspberries (fresh or frozen)
- 1 tbsp. low-carb maple syrup
- Optional: 2-4 ice cubes

Directions:

1. Add all the ingredients to a blender, including the optional coconut cream and ice cubes if desired, and blend for 1 minute.
2. Transfer the shake to a large cup or shaker, and enjoy!
3. Alternatively, store the smoothie in an airtight container or a mason jar, keep it in the fridge, and consume within 2 days. Store for a maximum of 30 days in the freezer and thaw at room temperature.

Forest Fruit Blaster (vegan)

Preparation time: 5 minutes

Cooking time: 0 minute

Servings: 4

Nutritions:

- Calories: 275kcal
- Fat:24.8g
- Protein: 8.5g
- Net carbs: 4g
- Fiber: 1.9g
- Sugar: 3.4g

Ingredients:

- ¼ cup mixed berries (fresh or frozen)
- ½ kiwi (peeled)
- 2 cups full-fat coconut milk
- 2 scoops organic soy protein (vanilla flavor)

- ½ cup water
- Optional: 2 ice cubes

Directions:

1. Add all the ingredients to a blender, including the optional ice if desired, and blend for 1 minute.
2. Transfer the shake to a large cup or shaker, and enjoy!
3. Alternatively, store the smoothie in an airtight container or a mason jar, keep it in the fridge, and consume within 2 days. Store for a maximum of 30 days in the freezer and thaw at room temperature.

Lemon Mousse

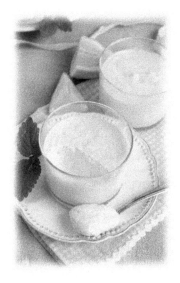

Preparation time: 10 minutes

Cooking time: 0 minute

Servings: 2

Nutritions:

- Calories 444
- Fat 45.7g
- Carbohydrates 10g

- Sugar 6g
- Protein 4.4g
- Cholesterol 0mg

Ingredients:

- 14 oz coconut milk
- 12 drops liquid stevia
- 1/2 tsp lemon extract
- 1/4 tsp turmeric

Directions:

1. Place coconut milk can in the refrigerator for overnight. Scoop out thick cream into a mixing bowl.
2. Add remaining ingredients to the bowl and whip using a hand mixer until smooth.
3. Transfer mousse mixture to a zip-lock bag and pipe into small serving glasses. Place in refrigerator.
4. Serve chilled and enjoy.

Avocado Pudding

Preparation time: 10 minutes

Cooking time: 0 minute

Servings: 8

Nutritions:

- Calories 317
- Fat 30.1g
- Carbohydrates 9.3g
- Sugar 0.4g
- Protein 3.4g
- Cholesterol 0mg

Ingredients:

- 2 ripe avocados, peeled, pitted and cut into pieces
- 1 tbsp fresh lime juice
- 14 oz can coconut milk
- 80 drops of liquid stevia

- 2 tsp vanilla extract

Directions:

1. Add all ingredients into the blender and blend until smooth.
2. Serve and enjoy.

Almond Butter Brownies

Preparation time: 15 minutes

Cooking time: 15 minutes

Servings: 4

Nutritions:

- Calories 82
- Fat 2.1g
- Carbohydrates 11.4g
- Protein 6.9g
- Sugars 5g
- Cholesterol 16mg

Ingredients:

- 1 scoop protein powder
- 2 tbsp cocoa powder
- 1/2 cup almond butter, melted
- 1 cup bananas, overripe

Directions:

1. Preheat the oven to 350 F/ 176 C.
2. Spray brownie tray with cooking spray.
3. Add all ingredients into the blender and blend until smooth.
4. Pour batter into the prepared dish and bake in preheated oven for 20 minutes.
5. Serve and enjoy.

Simple Almond Butter Fudge

Preparation time: 15 minutes

Cooking time: 0 minute

Servings: 8

Nutritions:

- Calories 43
- Fat 4.8g
- Carbohydrates 0.2g
- Protein 0.2g
- Sugars 0g
- Cholesterol 0mg

Ingredients:

- 1/2 cup almond butter
- 15 drops liquid stevia
- 2 1/2 tbsp coconut oil

Directions:

1. Combine together almond butter and coconut oil in a saucepan. Gently warm until melted.
2. Add stevia and stir well.
3. Pour mixture into the candy container and place in refrigerator until set.
4. Serve and enjoy.

Lightning Source UK Ltd.
Milton Keynes UK
UKHW020659130521
383647UK00001B/103